Pocket guide for first Aid treatments

I0438159

POCKET GUIDE

FOR FIRST AID TREATMENTS

STEP-BY-STEP GUIDANCE FOR EMERGENCY CARE

Philip kabcy PhD

Pocket guide for first Aid treatments

ISBN;13:978-1548309800
ISBN:10:154830980x

PUBLISHER NAME

McSndy publisher inc

Disclaimers

Knowledge and best practice in any field are constantly changing. As I research and experience broaden my knowledge, changes in practice, treatment, and drug therapy may become necessary. Readers are to check the most current information provided (a) on procedures featured and stated (b) by the manufacturer of each product to be administered, to verify the recommended dose or formula, the method and duration of administration, and contraindications if any. It is the responsibility of the practitioner, relying on their own experience and knowledge of the patient, to make diagnoses, to determine dosages and the best treatment for each individual patient, and to take all appropriate safety measures. To the fullest extent of the law, neither the Publisher nor the Author assumes any liab ity for any injury or property arising out or related to any use of the material contained in this book

Table of Contents

NOTE

First aid pocket guidance will arm you
knowledge that can save life.

NOTE

Introduction

Accident and emergency can be referred to any setting that requires immediate attention and care. Trauma is the causes of death and disability for the people aged from 1-55 years. The injury may be intentional or accidental about 2/3 total accident happen to be accidental while about 60% intentional injury are the causes of death, were due to the self-harm incidences.

Trauma injuries are the major causes of morbidity and mortality, as result blunt injuries and penetration by forceful impact in the body. All injuries by definition produce direct pressure damages, nature, and intensity dependent upon the site that is being affected (Anatomic site).Victims may survive the initial impact that may develop from the injury. The destruction of the blood vessel may lead to the loss of blood, which may either be internal or external bleeding.

This book will addresses the care on any emergency scene, site and situation which can be a working place or at home and during the occupational, terrorist attack. These conditions are required thorough evaluation and treatments conducted consecutively. Begin with systems that trigger the most immediately threatened to live if damage. It very essential for the caregiver to acquainted with basic principles of first aid treatment, emergencies preparedness, and common trauma management. It also a guide that would teach you various skill related to

17

accident and emergencies and disasters prevention. It makes you act like professionals during any emergencies situation so that to prevent the fatal mistake that might endanger victims life. For instance attending an injury to the leg or fractures alone, not considering the most important aspect of attending to dramatics life threat such obstruction of the airway can be a very dangerous mistake.

Evaluating and assessment of victim during first aid treatment is very crucial, to understand the mnemonic for easy to remember. These are the basic principles that can help you in all emergencies. These term as follows,(A, B, C, D) of emergency, is a systemic method of identity, triaging and rapidly examined for the major abnormalities,

18

knowledge of this is very necessary in order to be able to render first aid treatment perfectly.

First aid kit equipment

These kit contents should be kept in a clean, dry, airtight bag. Do not keep the container in a damp atmosphere place such as a bathroom and make sure that it is clear-labeled (FIRST AID BOX)

An emergency kit will help you to provide emergency and treatment in an efficient way.The contents of an emergency bag will vary considerably according to a place of practice.The proximity of a primary health center, medical clinic or hospital, your individual preference for practice in a specialty area only. standing orders for administration of medicines, injections, or any other treatment in an emergency.To add or delete items from the comprehensive list of suggested items given in the following section.

The emergency kit should be a portable divided with menus and pockets with flaps. Replacement of each item as soon as possible after use is imperative to avoid wasting time looking for items in an emergency. Check the kit regularly replenish when necessary and keep items in the same place at home or inside your car.

Emergency Kit Contents

1. Flashlight, (Medical use)
2. Assessment Tongue spatula
3. Thermometer
4. Aneroid sphygmomanometer

5. Stethoscope

6. Bandages, assorted sizes
7. Care Treatment Bandage triangular
8. Gauze pads, individually packed, sterile
9. Adhesive dressing strips (band-aid)
10. Cotton tipped applicators
11. Cotton wool, small packet
12. Adhesive tape
13. Safety pins, assorted sizes 1 dozen
14. Eye pads
15. Splints, light wood, plywood
16. Bottles, screw-topped, wide-mouthed (for specimen)
17. Catheters, plastic or rubber, urethral

18. Gastric lavage tube, rubber, medium size
19. Tourniquet or rubber tubing strip
20. Intravenous drip set, disposable type with needle
21. Hypodermic syringe - 2 ml.

Hypodermic syringe - 5 ml.

Hypodermic needles No.26, 24, 22 sizes

22. File for cutting ampoules
23. Pocket knife
24. Scalpel
25. Scissors blunt tipped
26. Scissors sharp pointed
27. Forceps, artery clamps
28. Forceps, dissecting
29. Dextran or Dextrose solution (as intravenous drip a starter in non-breakable flask or bag) 500 ml.

30. Oral Rehydration power

31. Tetanus Toxoid 5 ml.

32. Injection Adrenalin 1:1000 1 ml.

33. Injection Pethidine 100 mg in 2 ml.

34. Injection Morphine Sulphate 30 mg in 2 ml

35. Injection Morphine Sulphate 30 mg in 2 mls

36. Injection Atropine Sulphate 1 mg in 1 ml.

Combined Injection Morphine Sulphate and Atropine Sulphate

Oral Medications

- ➢ Antihistamines eg. Tablet Avil, Phenergan, Benadryl.

- ➢ Antispasmodics eg. Tablet Spasmindon, Belladonna

- Antiemetics eg. Tablet Sequel, Stemetil,
- Analgesics eg. Tablet Aspirin, Crocin, Paracetamol, Novalgin
- Anti-asthmatics eg.Tablet Aminophylline, Ephedrine
- Antacid eg. Tablet Aludrox, Gelusil

Topical Medications for External Application

- Rectified Spirit 30 ml.
- Tincture benzoin 30 ml.
- Tincture Iodine, weak
- Lotion Calamine 30 ml.
- Lignocaine/Xylocaine Ointment 9%
- Eye Oinment
- Tetracycline Eye Ointment 1%

Qualities of the first aider

The first aider requires these qualities.

1. He should have the basic and technical knowledge

2. He must be sympathetic and understanding the situations

3. He must use a logical sense of initiation quality as well as sense of leadership

4. He should have the ability to make decision quickly and decisively

5. He must know the limit of his intervention, that the less interference the better.

Principles of first aid management

1. He must be very vigilant and protect himself first.

2.   Treat the most urgent condition first, in order of priority (if the victims have the infection, bleeding and pain respectively. Considered to manage the bleeding first, prevent infection while pain treated lastly.

3.   Do your best to remove the victims from the source of danger or a danger from the victims.

4.   An unconscious victim is placed in recovery position i.e prone position with a head turn to one side.

5.   An unconscious victim and those who are vomiting or bleeding should never be given anything to drink by mouth.

6.   Alcoholic stimulant should never be given so, to avoid vital center depression in the brain.

7.   Reassure the victim

8.   Seek medical aid when necessary

9.   Organize unskilled crowd or survivor to help in any ways possible, they can be used to call an emergency number.

10.   Control crowd and prevent them from exiting the victims

11.   Handle the victim properly and gently. particularly if there is suspected fracture. In this case, you should support the affected limb with other opposite limbs.Do not lift the affected part unless you have sufficient helpers.

12.   Proper assessment of the situation is needed and very vital, especially if a decision is to be made regarding the need for the victim, medical aid or transportation to the heath care facilities.

Purpose of first aid management

1. To keep the victim alive

2. To prevent worsening of victim condition

3. To alleviating suffering and sustain life

4. To maintain life

Skill require for first aid workers

1. To identify the difference between life and death

2. To identify the possible disability of victim

3. To recognize the various stage of recovery

4. Triage and assess the situation quickly

5. He must be equipped with principles of first aid management

6.   To apply the basic principles to save the life at any given time when the injury occurs and ability to carried out various techniques at anywhere.

7.   Ability to recognizes and provide any material that can be improvised and use to prevent further victims suffering that sustain his life.

8. Ability to monitor vital signs, which are very crucial in the part of maintaining healthy continuum.

9. To be able to comprehend of symptom, history of the accident and secure the casualty from bystanders crowd.

10.   Ability to handle a casualty without adding unnecessary discomfort or pain and could effectively utilize appliances accurately, quickly and neatly.

EMERGENCY CARE

Emergency care is very demanding due to the versatility and diversity of it is different types,natures, degrees, conditions, and situations that warrant considering safety and risk management. The challenges include issues of occupational hazard risk that involve in it is a context of providing holistic and individualistic care to the accident victims.With regard to fast-paced technology driven environment, in which serious accident, trauma, illness could be encountered and confronted daily basis.

The dimension of the management disasters and terrorism which result to the mass casualty and destruction of lives and properties. While on the other hand the emergent of chemical and biological weapons. This situation necessitated that not only the emergency teams but also all the citizen must have extensive knowledge for first aid management and diseases prevention.

This encompasses recognition and treatment of individual exposed to all types of accidents range from minor skin abrasion to the higher level of mass casualty, which includes terror attack.The anticipation for the emergency care and respond in an event this need can never be overemphasized.

SECTION ONE

SCOPE AND PRACTICE OF EMERGENCY

The management of accident and emergency is a critical care given to the victims, that required urgent triage system that has been recognized and includes that concept of the emergency.It is considered for whatever the individual, family conspires it to be. Peoples seek emergency care for life-threatening disease such heart problems.The conditions such as cardiac arrest, angina pectoris and myocardial infarction, acute heart failure and cardiac arrhythmia, these require specializing education, training, and experiences to identify such types of urgent response from the first aider.

To be able to expertise in setting priority, identification of victim health problems are the essentials part of the first aider.Furthermore, an accurate establishment of triage is important for setting priorities, monitors and continuously assessing the accident victim.

Triage

Triage is a process of assessing victim health status so to determine the best management priorities.This priority can be urgent and non-urgent.This classification is based on the type of the need that victim requires.Urgent cares are the condition that needs serious illness, a trauma that if not treated quickly and immediately can result to life-threatening which might cause loss of life or permanent disability.Obstruction of the airway is an example of urgent treatment.The non-urgent category is a triage that indicates minor injury or illness in which the treatment may be delayed for some hours and this delay may not increase victim suffering and morbidity.

HEALTH RISK AND SAFETY

All emergency providers should strictly adhere and observe the universal standard precaution so that to minimize exposure.Due to the increased risk of exposure to infected blood with hepatitis B and Hiv.the first aid worker should safely observe the precaution, the health safety act provides structure for all modern health safety legislation.The foundation act placed a duty of responsibility on the state to the emergency team to cover their life insurance. The principle of self-safety is very imperatives for the rescue teams to protect them self first. They must have an eagle's eye, high sense of logical reasoning in a delivery of their services. The use of personal protective equipment and ability to improvise at the accident scene is important.

SYSTEMIC APPROACH TO EMERGENCY

Systemic ways of establishing and setting priorities for the victim with an emergency needs and health problems which comprise stabilization, prompt assessment, and treatment. The health priority includes primary survey and secondary survey.

Pain

Before describing these surveys, we would explain the chief complaint. The Pain is the sixth vital sign and one of the most common patient symptoms that encounter during emergencies, whether it be at home, or out home. The first aider role's in preventing pain is pivotal and cannot be underestimated. It requires many skills and techniques beyond simply given pain killer.Pain is an intensively personal and subjective phenomenon and only the patient knows what pain he is feeling. It influenced by a range of factors of which physiology is one. Other include psychological, contextual, environmental, social, cultural factors all interplay with individual's personality, previous experience, and health problems to affect the pain experience in a way that is unique to each person.

General approach to pain management

This is based on detailed history and thorough physical examination, assess the severity and degree of disability using pain score system. A plan is made of the modalities of the treatment to use,

37

and in which order, depending on the victims' respond.This book comprises a comprehensive step-by- step guidance for first aid management

Primary survey

The primary survey is regarded as urgent care to victims by quickly assessing and prompt stabilization of any life-threatening or disease condition.The mnemonic of this urgent cares is (A, B, C, and D).

A ---Airway patency

The normal respiratory air passage can be narrowed or threatened by the blood clot in the oropharyngeal and soft tissue laxity, this can easily be visible on direct inspection of the mouth. When patiently speaks can improve the airway patency, but when this clot goes down to the lower airway is very dangerous and catastrophe to the victim to survive if urgent care is not established quickly.blood and foreign body material can be removed by suction or manually.

1. Ensures that patient airway established

2. Provide adequate ventilation, cardiopulmonary resuscitation may be employed

3. Evaluate breathing, restore cardiac out through controlling of hemorrhage, preventing, treating shock, maintenance and restoring circulation.

B---Breathing

Ventilation is control by the respiratory center in the medulla oblongata of the brain, it may reduce respiratory drive when depressed. Inadequate air exchanges are usually apparent on auscultation.A condition such as tension pneumothorax, multiples rib fracture, pulmonary contusion may cause the deviation of the trachea to the side opposite to the injury.This can be identified by the decrease in breath sound, some time distension of neck vein and increase venous pressure.Inadequate ventilation is treated with endotracheal intubation and mechanical ventilation.

C---Circulation

External bleeding can occur from major blood vessel but this type of bleeding is likely apparent. internal bleeding may be life-threatened because of it often less obvious, however, the volume can occur in only few body compartment such as chest, abdomen and soft tissue in the pelvic.during assessment the pulse rate and blood pressure, the sign of shock noted.Dusky color, diaphoresis, altered mental status.When palpate the abdominal distension, tenderness, pelvic instability.internal bleeding requires exploratory laparotomy while external bleeding can be controlled by direct pressure.

D---Disability

The assessment of neurological functions is evaluated especially when suspecting spinal and head injuries.Major deficit are involved due to the cord damage.This can be examined by using a Glasgow coma scale.this type of injury is managed by manual stabilization of head and neck with neck collar stabilizer. The patient " log rolled" on a side to allow examination.

Secondary survey

After primary survey has been established, the secondary survey consist

1.   Complete physical examination from head to toe

2.   Proper history taking from victim or relative, bystanders

3.   Laboratory diagnostic test

4.   Setting of monitor device such as ECG, catheter etc

5.   Splinting of suspected fracture, wound cleaning and sterile dressing

6.   Intervene base on victim condition

After immediate cares a thorough evaluation focused on obtaining further information using mnemonic "**AMPLE**" these cover essential data from the victim

A---Allergy

M---Medication

P---Past medical history

L---Last meal

E---Event of injury.

An open wound is covered with the sterile dressing, but cleaning and repair are deferred until completion of evaluation and treatment of more serious. Obvious suspected fracture is splinted pending on imaging.

TERRORISM AND DISASTER MANAGEMENT

In the world history, the human had suffered for various types of disasters which were resulted to million lives perished and hundred thousand suffered different types of disability.Mass casualty associated with a disaster, man-made terrorism, wars all over the world consumed human lives that were no been statistically noted. Warfares are not new in human history, but in the recent decades, the concept of weapons of mass destruction are widely spoken in the media.The WMDS term was dated back as six century BC and for biological and chemical weapons were dated back as 436 BC.

Today the rate of terrorism has in the increasing rate world widely.terroris are more sophisticated, equipped and well organized than the past.The availability of technology has is on side of the coins.the Oklahoma City bombing of Marah building in 1995, the bombing of world trade center towers and damage of Pentagon on September 11, 2001. In the same year, biological Anthrax exposure is open the new chapter of the world terrorism. The question is not whether it will happen, but when it will happen again, the recent terrorist attack in London signify that it is necessary for all to be aware and have the basic emergency skill, knowledge terror preparedness.

PREPEREDINESS

All nation must prepare for the way to protect it's citizen, organized effective emergency response system.Basically, early detection, protection, containment, and prevention.Decontamination of biological and chemicals agent that might result to havoc to the individuals, community as well as the environment.This agent after being incubated over the period of time can result in the epidemic.The following are some of the principles of awareness.

1.   Awareness of an unusual increase incident of fever, or respiratory and gastrointestinal complaint

2.   Any large number of rapidly fatal cases should cause an alarm and raise

suspicious especially when the death occurs after 72 hours.

3.   Increases in disease incidence in a given population that were apparently healthy, this should also cause an alarm

4.   Increase vigilant and security awareness of self, individuals, neighborhood and report any suspicious motives, a movement to appropriate critical and stress management agency.

5.   Take note of any illness with unusual frequency in the year, cluster patients from single location should cause an alarm of suspicious.

The following are examples of the agent that can be used as biological weapons.

Biological weapons

Anthrax

An anthrax is a genus of bacteria called anthrax bacillus, naturally occurring gram positive, encapsulated rod shape, sporulated bacteria.When this spores release into the air and inhale or via contact with meat(infected meat) inhalations of this spore can result to infection.

It is scientifically belief that only the infective dose of such organism is from 8000 to 50,000 of that spores must be inhaled to put an animal or human at risk.The incubation period is about 60 days which make it very difficult to identify the source of bacteria.

Sign and symptom

A cough   mild chest discomfort

Headaches   dyspnoea

Fever   syncope without nasal congestion

Vomiting   Chill

Weakness

Treatment

Anthrax is penicillin sensitive organism, if the antibiotic begin within 24 hours after exposure, death may be prevented. the the drug of choice are;

1. Erythromycin

2.Chloramphenicol

3. Gentamicin

4.if the casualty are much ciprofloxacin, doxycycline is recommended.

Manage the victim under standard precaution.

Smallpox

Smallpox is a DNA virus with the incubation period of about 12 days. The organism is highly contagious and spread by direct contact with clothing, linen or droplet.This organism was used as biowarfare during the Franch and Indian War 1754-1756 when blanket from the smallpox patient was sent to India, that was the result of more than 50% mortality rate of that particular war.

Sign and symptom

High-grade fever

Malaise

Headaches

Backaches

Prostatitis

Maculopapular rashes

Treatment

Treatment include supportive care with antibiotic and the victim must be isolated using barrier method

Chemical weapons

Agents that can be used for chemical weapons are more volatile and more quickly than those caused by biological weapons. This chemical agent can be used by the terror group which can cause panic and social anxiety, these substances include those that affect nervous system, respiratory system, and vascular system. This agent can be converted to vapors, the most volatile among them are phosgene and cyanide.

1.Nervous system agent

Causes;

Sarin and soma organophosphate

Sign and symptom

Increase gastrointestinal motility

Diarrhea

Bronchospasm

Treatment

Clean body with soap and water

Decontamination

Benzodiazapham

Atrophin

2. Respiratory system agent

Cause;

Phosgene and chloride

Sign and symptom

Pulmonary oedema

Bronchospasm

Treatment

Airway management

Ventilation

Bronchoscopy

3.vascular system agent

Cause;

Cyanide

Sign and symptom

Tachypnea

Tachycardia

Respiratory arrest

Respiratory failure

Coma and seizure

Cardiac arrest

Treatment

Sodium nitrate

Sodium thiocyanate

Amyl nitrate

Hydroxyl cobalamin

Other substances that can be used are heavy metal, vesicant, volatile toxin.Example of this agent as follows

Arsenic, lead, benzene, chloroform, sulfur, and mustard.

SECTION TWO

CARDIOPULMONARY RESUSCITATION

The stages of resuscitation can be separated into three component, basic life support, and advanced life support. This section concentrates purely on basic life support.CPR is an organized, sequential response to cardiac arrest, including recognition of absent breathing and circulation, basic life support (BLS) with chest compressions and rescue breathing, advance cardiac life support(ACLS) with definitive airway and rhythm control, and post-resuscitative care.

Cardiac arrest

Cardiac arrest is the sudden cessation of the circulation in a person that is not expects to die at that time.

Characteristic features

1. Loss of consciousness
2. Absent of breathing (apnoea)
3. Absent of carotid pulse
4. Cyanosis

Absent of carotid pulse is the most reliable diagnostic features' absent of radial pulse is not diagnostic and the onset of cyanosis may be delayed.

Causes of cardiac arrest

Cardiac arrest may occur as in two forms;

Ventricular fibrillation in which the cardiac impulse is not regular at ventricles.while another form is asystole by which the impulse generation is impaired from the pacemaker.

1. Hypoxia

2. Massive haemorrhage

3. Myocardiac ischaemia

4. Severe cardiac disease

5. Severe vagal stimulation

6. Severe electrolyte disturbance e.g potassium and calcium

7. Pulmonary embolism

8. Severe cardiac dysrthmias

9. Electrocution

10. Drugs e.g myocardic depressant.

The chain of survival

The chain of survival consists of four links.If a victim has to the optimum chances of survival from cardiac arrest, then all the links of the chain must be present. These four links are as follows;

1. Early access
2. Early basic life support
3. Early defibrillation
4. Early advance life support

1. Early access.

Early access involves swift recognition of a cardiac arrest and the prompt activation of the emergency services.Assistance is obtained from via 999 system,

2. Early basic life support

Early basic life support is essential if the brain damage is to be prevented.Research has shown that without basic life support it takes 3-4 minutes for a patient to suffer irreversible brain damage after a collapse, or less if the patient was initially hypoxic.On more positive note, if good basic life support skills are applied, these can buy time for the arrival of a defibrillator.

3. Defibrillation

Defibrillation is one of the few resuscitation treatments proven to be effective, but it is success tend to depend on the time elapsed post collapse. Research has shown that patient's chances of survival after collapse from cardiac arrest decrees by 7-10% for every minute without defibrillation. Nowadays, the advent of easy-to-use defibrillation is available within the wider community and it becomes common at the public place such as airport and railway.

4.Early advance life support

Early advance life support involves the application of techniques that attempt to stabilize the patient's condition, the practical skill such as obtaining intravenous access, the administration of drugs and endotracheal intubation is all aspect of this.

TECHNIQUE OF CPR

When cardiac arrest occurs, prompt CPR is indicating to prevent brain damage or death.It divided into three phases;

A. Basic life support

B. Advanced life support

C. Prolonged life support

The steps involved in each phase is conveniently listed in the order of alphabet A to E

SUPPORT (BLS) BASIC LIFE

Airway maintenance

Breathing assistance

Circulation assistance

ADVANCE LIFE SUPPORT (ALS)

Drugs

Electrocardiogram (ECG)

Fibrillation treatment (defibrillation)

PROLONGED LIFE SUPPORT (PLS)

Gauging (assessment of salvageability)

Human stability (measures for cerebral recovery)Intensive care(multiple organs support).

When confronted with victims suspected cardiac arrest

1. Shake and shout to patient to established unconsciousness

2. Feel for carotid pulse to established cessation of circulation

3. Call for help, but stay with the patient

4. Start Basic life support

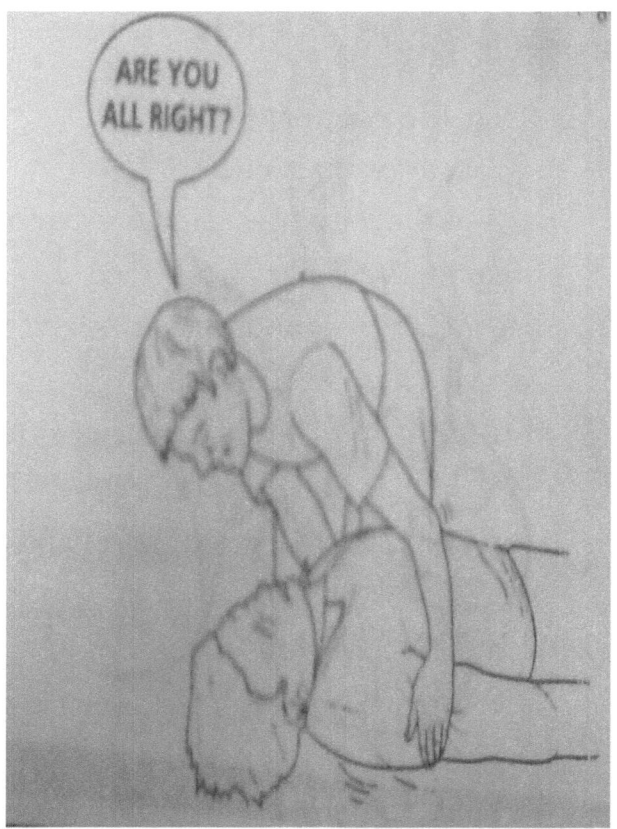

Fig 1 Establishment of cardiac arrest

Basic life support (BLS)

Airway maintenance

A patient airway is maintained by one or more of the following method depending on location, facilities, and experience;

1.   Backward head tilt (extension) with the chin pulled forward

2.   Use artificial airway oropharygeal or nasopharyngeal

3.   Tracheal intubation

4. Cricothyrotomy if all the above fail.

Valuable time should not be wasted in an attempting unfamiliar method, vomits or secretion must be cleared from the mouth.

Breathing assistance

Ventilation should be stated as soon as possible by one of the following methods as applicable.

1. Mouth to mouth breathing with the barrier(kiss of life)The operator stays on the right side of the patient, closes the nose with one hand, and breathes expired air into the patient's mouth. the chest must be observed to expand with each inflation

2. Mouth to nose breathing

The mouth is closed with one hand, and the operator breathes into the patient nose. This method is used when the operator's mouth is too small for the patient mouth.

3.Mouth to airway

The mouth breathes expired air through the special double-ended oral airway.

4.Mask and Bag

A facemask is applied over the patient mouth and nose and self-inflating bag(Ambu bag) is connected to the ventilator.

5.Endotracheal tube and bag

It the patient has an endotracheal tube in place, the tube is connected to the Ambu bag for manual ventilation. The fist method of choice is the one immediately available, and the one the first aider or operator is most familiar.

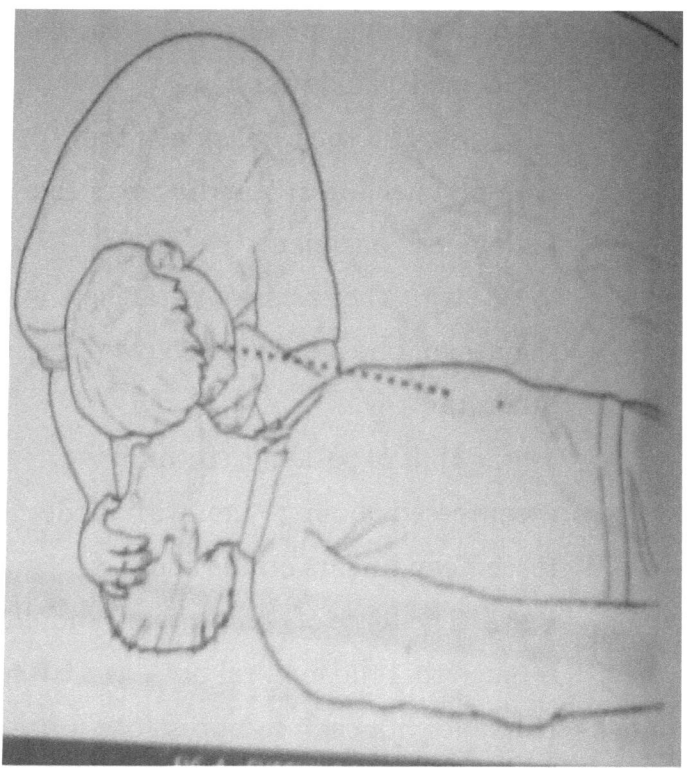

Fig 2 Breathing assessment

Circulation maintenance

The circulation should be re-established as soon as possible by external cardiac massage. This is performed as follows;

1.   Stay on the right side of the patient, kneeling or standing over the patient as convenient

2.   with both arms outstretched, and the heel of one hand cupped over the other, the low

3.   Half of patient's sternum is compressed about 4-5cm. with moderate force.Keep fingers on the chest.

4.   The force of compression should be such that the femoral pulse is palpable with each compression

5.   The weight of the body transmitted through the outstretched arm(elbow not bent) should be used rather than the arm muscles.

6.   The hands should not be completely lifted off the sternum

68

between compression, though pressure should be released.

7.   In small children, sternal compression should be done with only one hand, with gentle pressure on the middle of the sternum(the heart in children is higher in the chest than the adult)

Recommend rates of compression.

A.   For one operator; 15 compressions with 2 quick lung inflation

B.   For two operator;60 compressions with lung inflation interposed after every fifth compression.

NOTE;

Ensure safety

Approach any situation with extreme care, ensuring there is no danger primary to yourself, and secondary to the casualty. Hazard will very much depend on the situation in which you find yourself, but could include traffics,electricity, chemicals,animal, kichen implements, or falling masony etc.

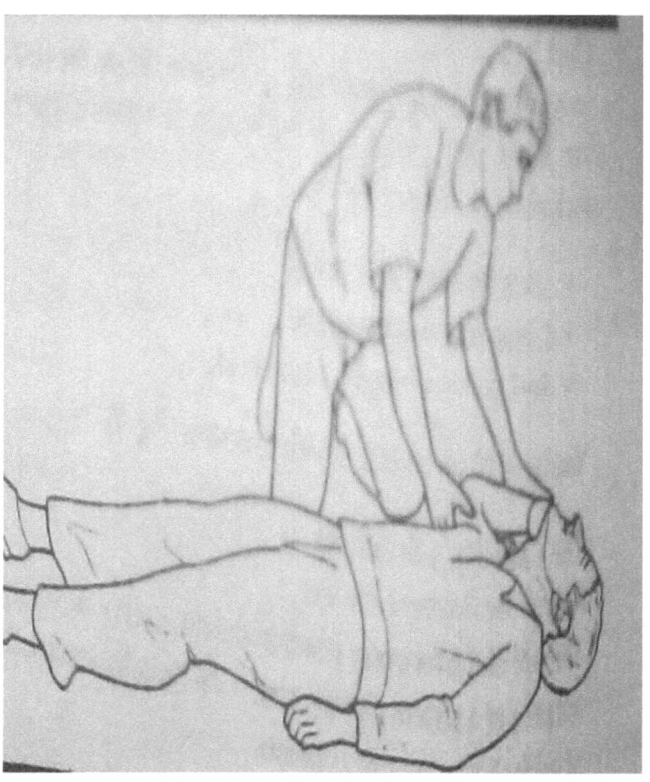

Fig 4 Check for breathing

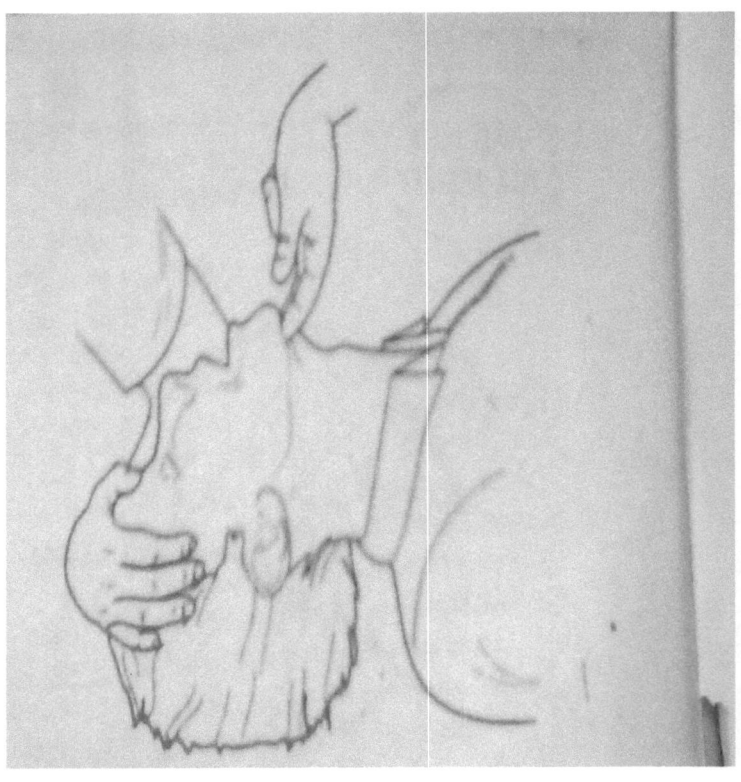

Fig 3 Opening of airway

Advanced life support(ALS)

This phase involve;

Drug

Electrocardiogram

Fibrillation treatment

Drugs

An intravenous line is established as soon as possible for the administration of drug and fluid.The drug commonly used can be easily remembered by the alphabets A, B,C,D as stated below.

A   for: Adrenaline 0.5-1 mg i.v repeated as necessary it increase cardiac contractility.

Atropine (.05-1 mg i.v)

B for: Bicarbonate (as dictate by the blood gases)

for: Correct metabolic acidosis. Monitor arterial gases

C for: Calcium chloride or gluconate(5-10 ml of 10% solution) if there is

Hypocalcaemia.This improves cardiac contractility.

D for: Dopamine (2-5 ug/kg/min as an infusion) this may be needed later to support the circulation once re-established and to improve renal blood flow.

Electrocardiogram(ECG)

This is useful in recognizing the types of cardiac rhythm, especially dysrhythmias this is important for appropriates treatment.

1. Asystole this can be treated with adrenaline or calcium

2. Ventricular fibrillation this is treated with DC shock.

Fibrillation treatment(defibrillation) indication

1. Ventricular tachycardia
2. Ventricular fibrillation

Electrode placement

The positive paddle is placed over the cardiac apex, the negative paddle is placed just below the right clavicle. Conductive jelly is applied to the paddle before placement.

Dose of direct current

Adult   : 400 joules

Children : 100-200 joules

Direct current(DC) is preferable to alternative current(AC), during application care should be taken to avoid physical contact with a patient or patient bed.

Treatment outcome of cardiac arrest

Following CPR, the heart my;

1. Recover without any brain damage

2. Recover with residual minor brain damage

3. Recover but with brain damage

4. Not recover (cardiac death)

SECTION THREE

Respiratory Emergencies

The respiratory emergency is any condition that interrupts the pulmonary gas exchange for more than 5 minutes and results to normal breathing stops or in which there is diminish oxygen saturation, intake is insufficient to support life.

Situations requiring airway control

1. Obstruction of the airway by the tongue when it is relaxing to close glottis.

2. Inhalation of a small amount of food, smoke, irritation, foreign body, and toxic chemicals, etc.

3. Compression of the neck by upper trauma

4. Respiratory disease such laryngospasm

5. Drowning

6. Strangulation and laryngeal edema

7. Combustible gases such carbon monoxide

Signs and symptoms

1. Apnea (unable to breath)

2. Loss of consciousness

3. General pallor (paleness)

4. Dyspnea (difficulty in breathing)

5. Respiratory failure

First Aid for Respiratory problem

1. Shout for help (depend on the condition)

2. Determine the consciousness of the casualty by tapping the victim on the shoulder and asking loudly "Are you ok!"

3. Assess and ensure that patient airway is clear and patent

4. Place the patient flat supine position with the head turned to one side

5. Remove any cloth around the neck that is preventing the taking in of air (Remove constraints from the neck)

6. Kneel at a right side of the patient's head placed one hand under his neck and the other hand under his lower Jaw extend his head and neck gently backward.This prevents the tongue from falling back into the throat.

7.   Place your cheek and ear close to the victim's mouth and Nose. Look at the chest to see if it rises, falls, and listen and fell for air to be exhaled for about 5 seconds.

8.   If the breathing is absent, pinch the victim's nostrils shut with thumb and index finger of your hand that is pressing on the victim's forehead.This action prevents leakage of air when the lungs are inflated through the mouth.

9.   Take a very deep breath and hold it.Fit your mouth tightly over the patient's open mouth and forcibly into the lungs.

10.   While carrying out artificial respiration, check the patient's pulse every 2 or 3 minutes to ensure the heart has not stopped.

11. Continue the breathing procedure at the rate 12 to 18 breaths per minute until the chest is up and the patient is breathing for himself or until is certain his is dead.

12. In children, our mouth should cover both his nose and mouth.Very gentle breathing should be used and the younger the child, this should continue at a rate of 25 breaths per minute.

Once the victims can breathe, place him in what is called the recovery position.

Check breathing

In order to check for breathing. Look in the mouth for foreign body(dentures can be left in place if they fit well). If anything is seen, remove it carefully. To

open airway perform a head
tilt/maneuver.

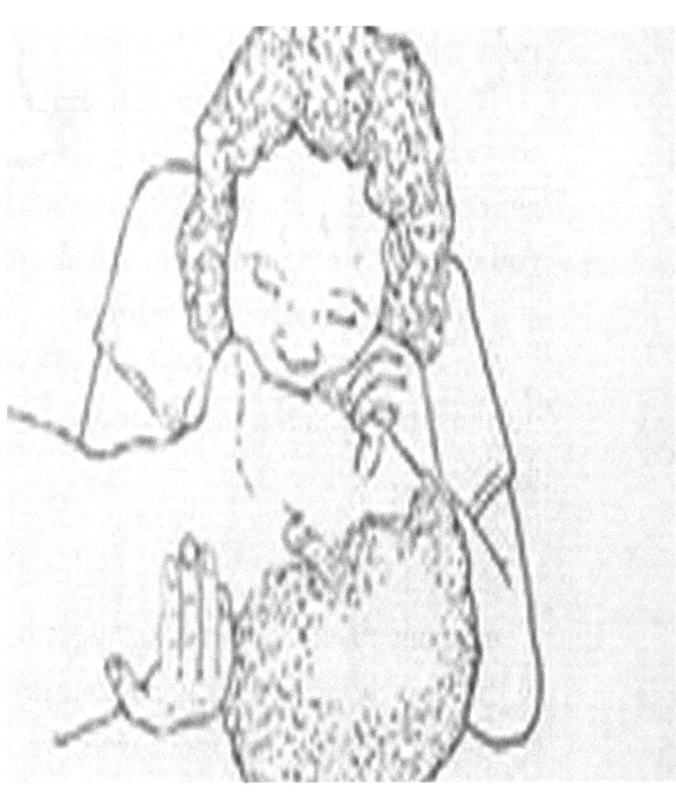

Fig. 5.How to give artificial respirtion

and positioning of casualty

1.   If mouth to mouth or mouth to the nose are failed and no pulse cardiopulmonary resuscitation is followed.(CPR) or heart-lung resuscitation is a combined effort to maintain circulation and breathing.

2.   CPR Is an emergency procedure applied when heart and lung actions have stopped.

Mouth to mouth respiration

(a) Airway can be blocked by the tongue,

(b) Clear airway by extending patient's head and neck;

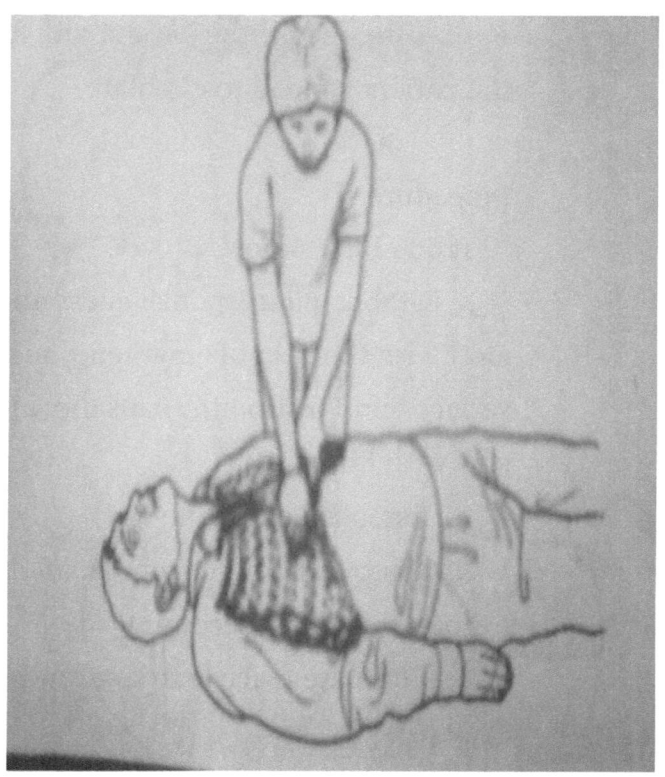

Fig.6 compression

For effective CPR you will have to

perform procedures to:

    1.   1.Create an open airway to

maintain circulation

2.   Breathe for the patient and force the patient's blood to circulate.

Procedure

If one First Aider

1. Establish unresponsiveness and alert with the help of emergency medical service and Position the causality and stay with him.

2. Establish patent airway.

3. Observe, Look, Listening, and feel for breathing (3-5 seconds).

4. Ventilate twice (1 to 2 seconds) per breath.

5. If no pulse (5-10 seconds)

6. Locate Compression site

7. Position your hands

8. Began compressions

9. Ventilate twice

10. Reassess pulse after 4cycles of ventilation, then every few minutes.

For two first aider rescuer CPR

1. Established and determine unresponsiveness

2. Ensure airway is open, look, listen, (feel 3-5 seconds)

3. Ventilate twice per breath (1 -2 seconds).

4. Determine no pulse and locate CPR compression site

5. Say "No pulse."Begin compressions

6. Ventilate once (1-2 seconds) Stop mouth-to-mouth ventilation.

7. Continue with one ventilation every 5 compressions.

8. After 10 cycles, reassess breathing and pulse.

No pulse says, "Continue CPR."Pulse-says, "Stop CPR." Assess for spontaneous breathing and pulse for 5 seconds at the end of the first minute, and few minutes thereafter.

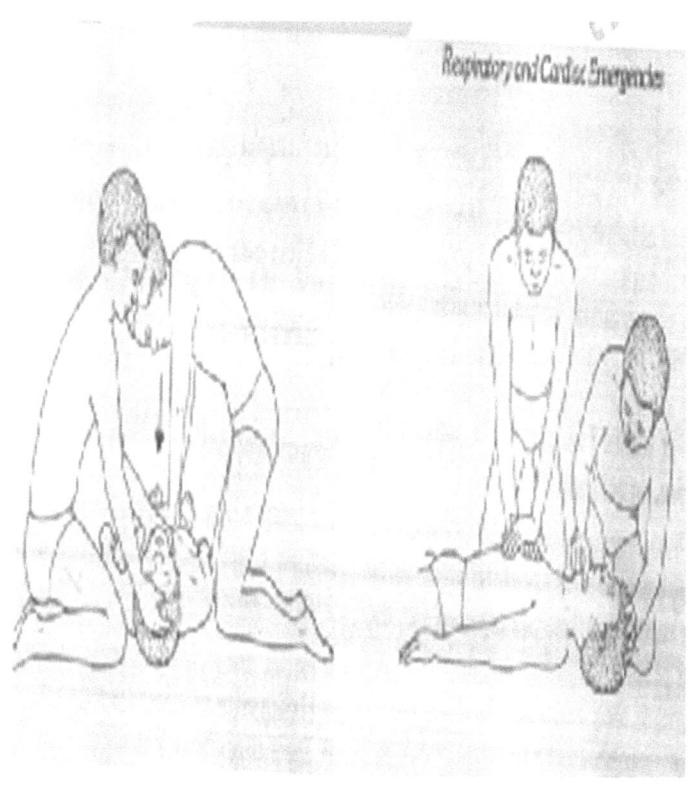

Fig. 7 Cardiopulmonary resuscitation by two first aider

Choking

Management of airway consist any techniques that pave to the clearance of airway.Maintenance open airway passage with the mechanical device and assisting respiration, when the equipment is not available, mouth to mouth ventilation is efficiently performed.When food or foreign body inhaled into the trachea when eating in which sometimes help is needed to assist the victims.

Heimlich maneuver

Heimlich maneuver is a thrust to upper abdomen is a preferred treatment for an awake choke. The techniques involve extending a (head lift) chin lift and thrusting the jaw forward.This maneuver stretches the anterior neck structure, lifting and drawing the tongue away from the back of the pharyngeal wall.Obstruction by foreign materials like dentures may be removed by finger swift, taking extreme care not to push it deeper.Do not make an attempt to hook the foreign body out with your fingers. This is likely to push it further down.

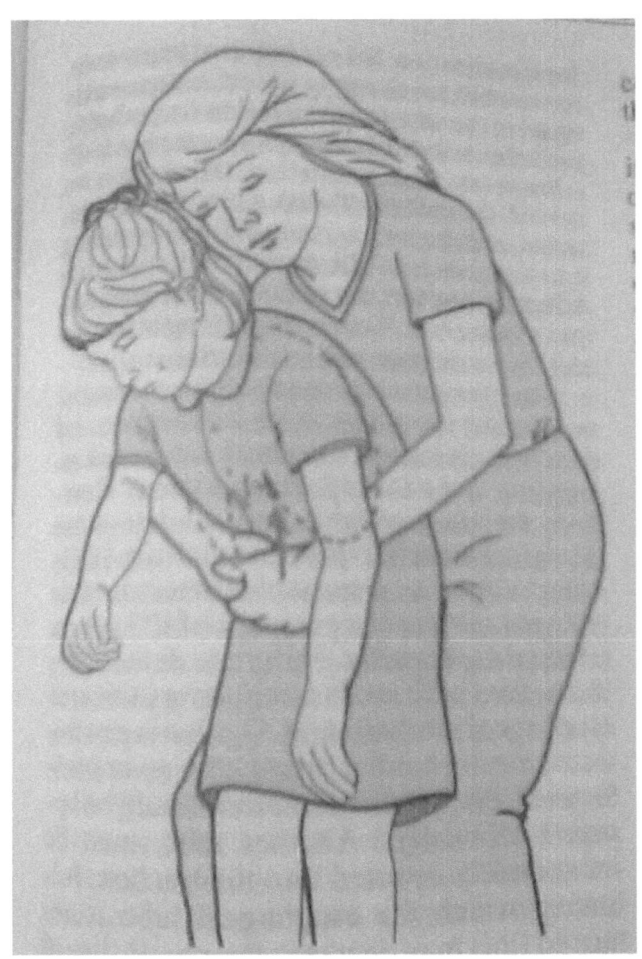

FIg.8 Abdominal thrush

For babies and small children:

Hold the baby upside-down by the feet and beat him/her timely between the shoulder blades.Lie the child face down over your knee or arm and beat them sharply between the shoulder blades.

In adults: there are two methods depending upon your knowledge and experience.

"Methods 1" stand erect behind the patient and hold around the chest just under the chest bone and give a short sharp hear hug

Fig.8 Method A removal of inhaled foreign body in adult

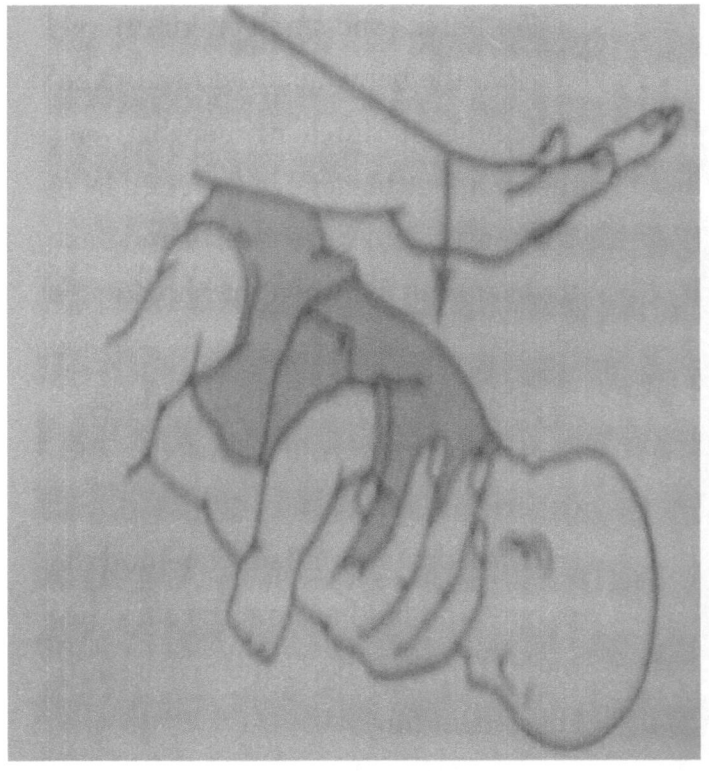

Fig. 9 Removal of inhaled foreign body
in a baby

"Method 2" The patient should lean over the back of a chair holding on to the seat and the tenanting him sharply 3 to 4 times between his shoulder blades.whatever the method you use the foreign body should be coughed out.

1. If the breathing has stopped, quickly begin mouth-to- mouth respiration

2. if you have done the above maneuvers, refer to the nearest hospital or health the Center.

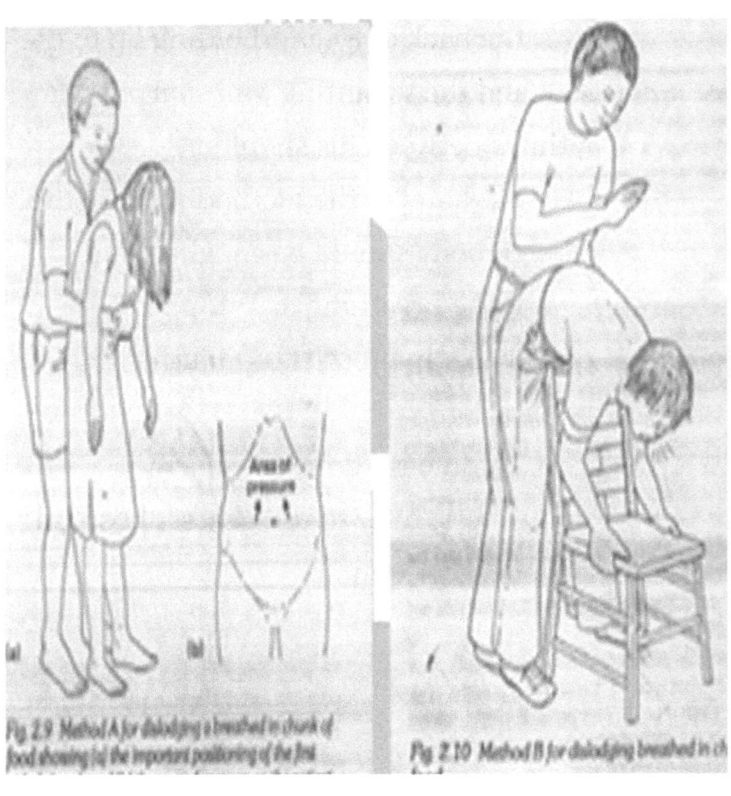

Fig. 10 Method 2

Drowning

When body immerse in water if the water reaches the lungs and either causing lung tissue damage or spasms of the airway that prevents the inhalation of air. Drowning is accidental suffocation in water, is the 7th most common cause of accidental death in the US overall and the 2nd most common cause in children ages 1-15 years. It can happen in many different places, Lake, swamp and spring, rivers.

Sign and symptom

1. Children may become submerged in less than one minute, more rapidly than adult may.

2. After rescue, a victim is anxiety, vomiting, wheezing

3. Respiratory failure

4. Tachypnea

5.Retraction and cyanosis

First Aid Management

1. Begin artificial respiration as soon as possible

2. You should not wait to get water out of the patient's chest first

3. If you cannot get air into his lungs, quickly turn the patient on his side, putting his head lower than the leg and push the body

4. Then give mouth-to-mouth artificial respiration.

5.If the condition of the patient is not improving refer the victim to the next health facility.

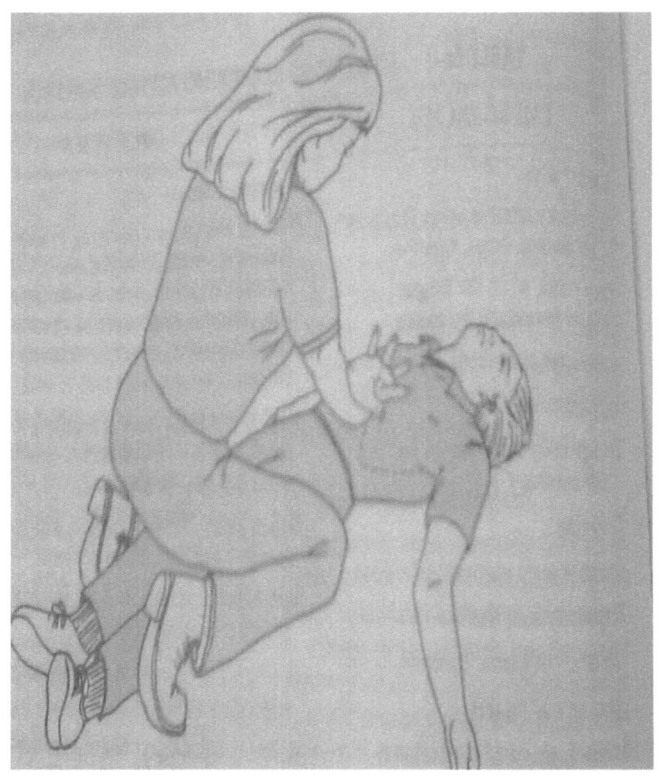

Fig.11 CPR in drowning victim

SECTION FOUR

Trauma

The injury is the number one cause of death in the world.There was 160,000 trauma associated death in the year 2003 in the US alone, the trauma can be categories as penetrating and blunt.

Penetrating injury comprises of any injury that breach the skin integrity by an object such as broken glass, knife or projectile types as the bullet and explosive.

The blunt injury involves a forceful impact such as kick, blow, fall, motor collision and blast.other types of the

100

injury includes thermal, chemical, toxic inhalation and ingestion, any injury that can result in tissues and organ damages are consider traumatic injury.

Wound

The wound is breaking in continuity to tissue of a body, it can either be internal or External.Depend on the nature and types of the wound the management might vary from debridement, closure with suture and exploration.The surrounding skin is cleaned, epidermal layers should not be exposed to hard chemical so that full strength substance like povidone iodine and hydrogen peroxide are avoided.

Classification of Wound

1.An open Wound is a break in the skin or mucous membrane

2.A closed wound is an injury to underlying tissue without a break external skin or mucous membrane.

Types of Wounds

1. Abrasion is a type of wound in which the is denuded

2. Incision is a wound that the edges' are regular

3. Lacerations is wound that has irregular edges

4. Punctures is an act of piercing with sharp object

5. Avulsions is the tearing of supporting structure

Causes of trauma

Cause or resulting in open wounds from:

1. Motor accidents

2. Fall

3. Mishandling of sharp objects, tools, and machinery

The main aims when dealing with trauma

1. Control the wound to stop bleeding

2. Treat and prevent shock

3. Prevent wound infection and contamination

4. prevent any complication

5. Seek medical attention when necessary

How Prevent wound infection

1. Hand washing before and after wound care.

2. Avoidance of contaminant

3. Use lean materials as much as possible E.g. cotton gauze, towels etc...

4. Wash in and around the victim's wound to remove bacteria and other dirty foreign material.

5. Wash the wound thoroughly by flushing with clean water, but preferably running tab water is better.

6. Apply sterile clean dressing and bandage the wound secure it firmly in place, Small wounds even can be taken care at home

7. If there is present of infection refer the victim to the health center

Hemorrhage

Stopping hemorrhage is an essential to the care and survival of victims during emergency and disaster situation.Excessive bleeding lead to the reduction of blood volume in circulation is the main cause of shock.Minor bleeding which is mainly from the veins, this type generally can stop spontaneously.

Types of bleeding

1.   Arterial bleeding is bright red in color due to presence of oxygen, flow from the wound inside

2. Venous bleeding is dark red in color due to lack of oxygen, flow is steady

3. Capillary bleeding is oozing from a bed of capillaries, red in color, usually less bright due to low oxygen saturation, than arterial blood with slow flow.

Methods of controlling bleeding externally

1. Rapid assessment of the bleeding site and patient clothing cut away.

2. Identify the area of bleeding

3. Direct pressure can be applied using compressed against the bleeding

4. Pressure bandage can be placed to hold pads of cloth. Put a thick pad of cloth held between the hand

5. Elevation an injured part of the body and it should be raised about the victim's heart.

6. Applying pressure on the supplying artery especially on extremity to minimizes severe bleeding.

6. Apply tourniquet in severe and tagged T to the victim so that to identify the time of applying.

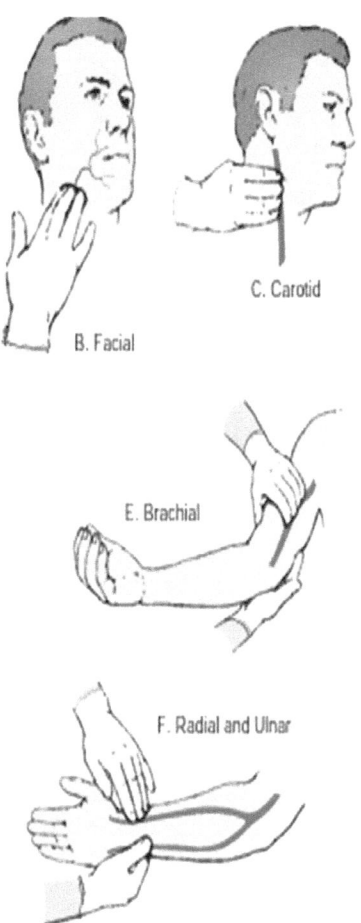

B. Facial

C. Carotid

E. Brachial

F. Radial and Ulnar

Fig 12. Pressure points for controlling bleeding

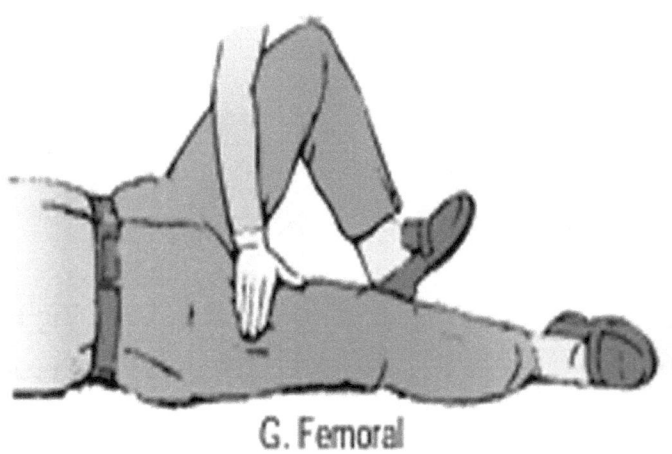

G. Femoral

P[71.2 Pressure points for control of hemorrhage

Fig 13 femoral pressure point for
controlling internal bleeding

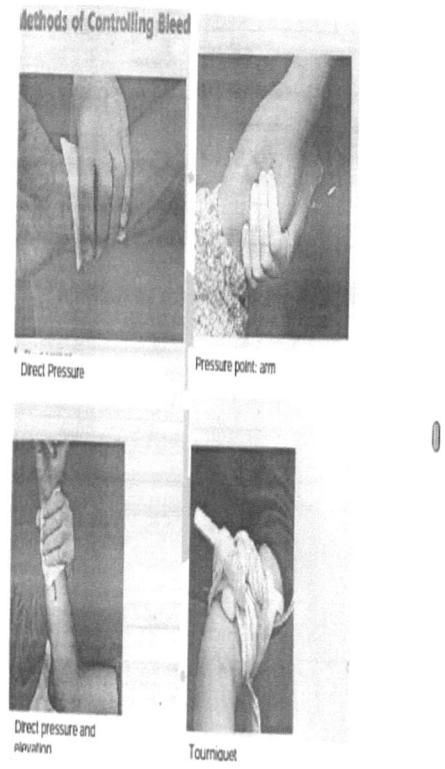

Fig.14Methods of controlling Bleeding

1. Direct pressure and elevation
2. Tourniquet

3. Pressure point: arm

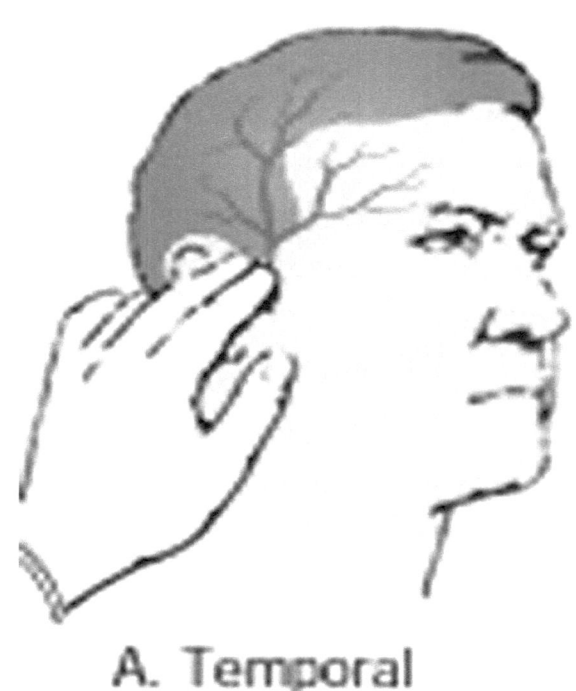

A. Temporal

Fig 15 temporal pressure point

Management of internal bleeding

1. Sign of shock is indicated possible internal bleeding

2. Resuscitate the victims and insert two large-bore canular

3. Start fluid replacement of isotonic electrolyte solution e.gRinger's lactate

4. Maintains circulation

5. Blood sample obtain for crossmatch and ABO types

6. Packed cell RBC infused when there is massive bleeding.

Shock

Shock is a dynamic clinical syndrome usually characterized by hypotension and inadequate tissues perfusion, with resultant metabolic acidosis, oliguria and altered level of consciousness.This reaction of the body to the failure of the circulatory system to provide enough blood to all the vital origins of the body.

Types of shock

A.   Hypovolemic shock

Cause; hypovolaemic may result from

1.   Internal and external blood loss

2.   Plasma loss in burns

3.   Electrolyte and water loss in severe diarrhea or vomiting

B.   Cardiogenic shock

1.   Acute myocardial infarction

2.   Severe cardiac dysrhythmias

3.   Severe cardiac diseases

C.   Septic shock

1.   This usually results from severe sepsis, especially gram-negative sepsis that is associated with bacterial

endotoxin.e.g E.coli,klebsiella and Pseudomonas

2. Gram positive organism includes staphylococci and streptococci

D. Neurogenic shock

This is the often results from spinal and cord injury, there is the loss of vasomotor tone causing widespread peripheral vasodilatation and hypotension but the blood volume is normal.

E. Anaphylactic shock

Anaphylactic shock may result from

1. Drug reaction(e.g penicillin)

2. Animal vaccine

3. Insect bites

4. Some food product

Sign and Symptoms of shock

General body weakness – the most significant symptoms

1. Nausea with possible vomiting
2. Thirst
3. Dizziness
4. Restlessness, and fear sign of shock
5. Fast breathing and shallow
6. pulse – rapid and weak
7. Pupils - dilated
8. Face – pale
9. Lips-blue, Restlessness, become unresponsive
10. Skin- cool and clammy- eyes- lackluster
11. Breathing – rapid and shallow

First aid management of shock

1. Position the patient lie down and stay at rest

2. Keep the airway patent and preventing the forward tilting of the head

3. Manage external bleeding

4. Keep the patient warm by covering with blanket or sheet so to prevent hypothermia

5. place the patient properly to assume anatomical position

6. Open airway and observe possible for vomiting

If there is no spinal injuries use one of the following positions, elevate the lower extremities, place patient place patient-flat, face up, and elevate the legs 8 to 12 inches.

1. you should not tilt the patient's body

2. Do not elevate any fractured limb unless they have been properly splinted

3. Should not elevate the leg if there are fractures to the pelvic

4. Do not give anything by mouth (NPO)

5. Monitor the patient vital signs such as pulse, respiration, blood pressure etc.

6. Refers the victim to the nearest health center.

Unconsciousness

The patient is said to be unconscious when he asleep, cannot speak and has no control over his movement.The victim is not oriented to place, people and time (PPT).

117

Cause of unconsciousness

1. Head and spinal injury
2. Fainting and Downing
3. Heart attack or block
4. Asphyxia
5. Poisoning
6. Shock
7. Epilepsy
8. Diabetic coma

Aim of the first aid management

1. To rule out the cause of the condition and manage it as quickly as possible and refer to Hospital.

Level of unconsciousness grade

1. Alertness: Patient can speak, answers, alert, questions and feels pain

2. Lethargy: Patient is awake but answers questions slowly and he may be confused about what is happening and where he is.

3.   Drowsiness: the patient is not asleep and is unable to concentrate on what we are saying

4.   Semi-consciousness: the patient is very sleepy of and has great difficulty in speaking and in answering your questions

5.   Unconsciousness: the patient is sleepy we cannot be able to speak and has no control his movements

Treatment of unconscious Patient

Principles of the treatment   A,B,C,D, i.e.

A--Assessing airway

B-- Check breathing

C--Check circulation using or by taking Vital sign

D-- Check for any bleeding and attempt to stop bleeding

119

1.   If the victim is improving lie in Recovery position

2.   Should not give an unconscious victim anything by mouth

3.   Establish level of responsiveness, using Glasgow Coma scale, check pulse, breathing rate and record any observations

4.   Prioritize to respiratory problems and heartbeat.

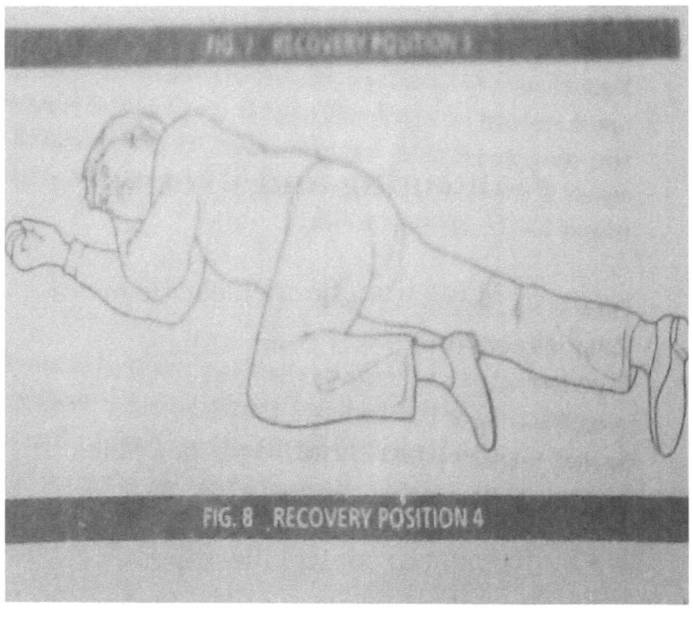

Fig. 16. Recovery position of an
unconscious patient.

SECTION FIVE

Bandaging and Dressing

Made from flannel, elastic net or special paper cotton cloths

Bandages are used for:

1. Hold splint in proper place

2. Maintain direct pressure over dressing to control bleeding.

3. Retain dressings and splints in position

4. Prevent or reduce swellings

5. Restrict movement and use sterile material

6. Bandage should never be used directly on a wound alone

7. Bandaging a wound should be applied firmly enough to keep dressing

122

and splints in position without too much pressure

Types of bandages

1. Triangular bandages
2. Roller gauze bandage
3. Elastic bandage
4. T- blinder bandage
5. Many-tailed abdominal bandage
6. Bandage should not be tight, it may cause injury to the part or impair circulation of blood, Lose bandage is also useless

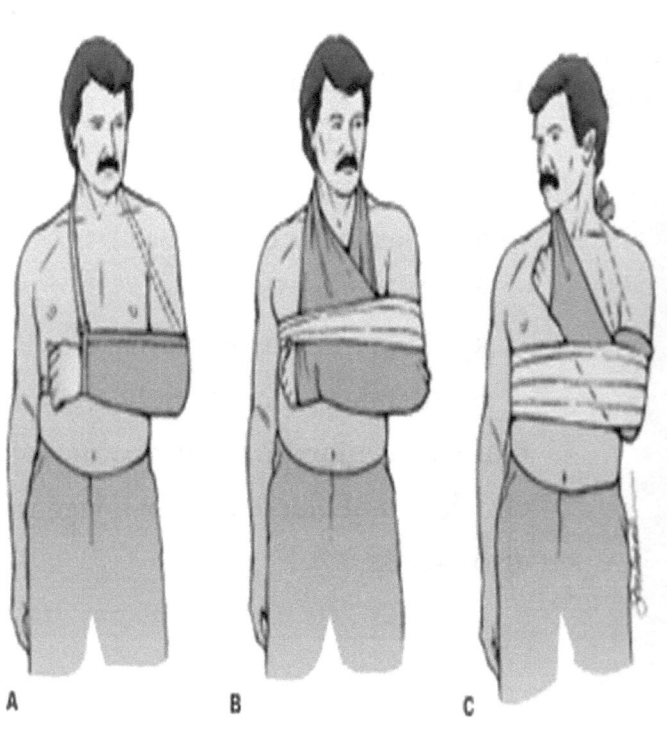

Fig 17. Types of bandages

Dressings

A dressing is a sterile protective covering applied to a wound to:

1. Prevent infection
2. Absorb discharge
3. Control bleeding
4. Avoid further injury
5. An efficient dressing should be sterile (germ-free) with the high degree of porosity and allow for oozing of discharge of fluid.

Fracture

The fracture can be described Is a crack of bone tissue or discontinuation of bone tissue due to different causes or accidents.

cause:

1. Accident or trauma

2. pathological due to bone infection

3. Tumor of the Bone

Types of Fracture

1. Closed

2. Open

3. compound/complicated

Signs and symptoms of fracture:

1. Protruding of the parts

2. Swelling

3. Crepitation

6 Splint fractures

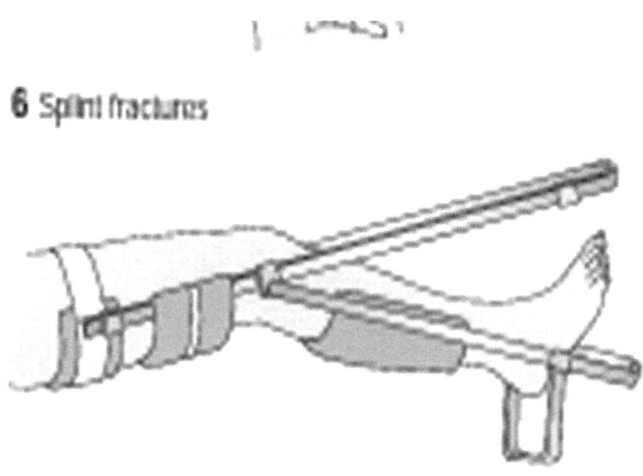

Fig. 19 Immobilization of spine fracture with traction

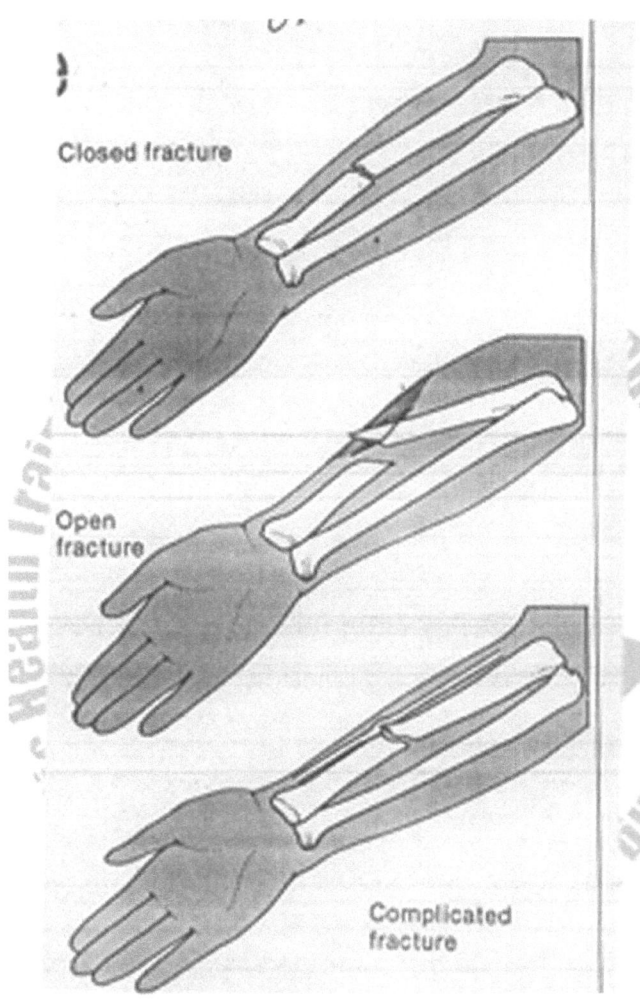

Fig.18. Types of fractures.

4. Deformity

5. Abnormal motion and unable to function

6. Numbness or tingling sensation

7. Patient may shout due to severe pain

8. Discoloration (ecchymosed)

Complications fracture

Immediate complications

1. Hemorrhage/ bleeding

2. Severe pain

3. Shock due to bleeding

Late complications of fracture

1. Disability

2. Disfiguring

3. Deformity

4. Malunion or non-union

5. Delay in Union

General First Aid management of Fracture

1. Assess victims carefully but very fast

2. Check respiratory status

3. Check bleeding thoroughly

4. Estimate the amount of blood loss

5. Determine and arrange for referral

6. Asphyxia, bleeding, and severe wounds must be dealt urgently.

7. Before treating any fracture Support the injured part with supporting device, immobilize the fracture, bandaging and use splints

8. Refer the victims to hospital urgently

Proper immobilization is essential in preventing further trauma, pain, and complications.

Dislocation

Dislocations are complete separation of the bone that are articulated to form joint or when a bone is no more in an anatomical position and the displacement of one or more bone at a joint.

Cause:-

1.   Strong force pull directly or indirectly on a joint

2.   Sudden muscular contraction of muscles

Most frequently dislocated are shoulder, elbow, thumb, finger, Jaw.

Signs and symptoms

1.   Pain, near the joint, victim cannot move it,

2. Deformity and abnormal appearance.

3.   Swelling is usually present

First aid and manage of dislocation

1.   Support and secure the part in most comfortable position

2.   obtain medical aid at once

3.   You should not make any attempt to replace the bones to normal position

4.   It is quite similar to the fracture.

5.   Do not delay to refer victims with fracture or dislocation since proper investigation and management is done at hospital

Strain and Sprain

Strain

The tear may occur in ligament is called sprain while in the muscle is strain overstretching of muscles due to over pulling of muscles.

Causes:

1. Lack of pre- exercise before doing any active sport

2. Lifting of heavy loads

3. Lifting of heavyweight

4. The common one is back strain.

Signs and symptom

toms Pain (sudden pain at the site of the injury)

1. Stiffness of muscles at the joint

2.   Difficulty in moving the affected joints

Management and First Aid of sprain and strain

1.   Get the victim in the most comfortable position

2.   Cold compress during fracture phase to increase vasoconstriction

3.   Warm compress (physiotherapy) to increase vasodilatation

4.   support and elevate the injured part or limb and give analgesia

5.   If not improved refer the victim

6.   In case of back strain use a hardboard under the bed or lay the victim down on a firm surface

Sprain

An injury which occurs as result of damages to the ligaments and tissue around particular joints are suddenly twisting or tearing.When the tear in minimal is referred as 1st degree, moderate 2nd degree and severe 3rd degree.

1.   A sprain is more severe than strain due to disruptions of tendons.

2.   Usually, it happens or occurs at joint especially at ankle joint.

3.   It might involve bone (broken)

4.   Sprain is also tendon defect

Signs and symptoms

1.   Pain especially on movement

2.   Swelling and tenderness

3.   Loss of movement and joint instability

Treatment: All tears treatment includes (RICE)

Rest, Ice, Compression, and Elevation

1.   Apply a cold compress

2.   Renew the compressed when they get warm and dry

3.   Support the joint in comfortable position with bandage

4.   Bandage firmly and securely with figure of eight bandage

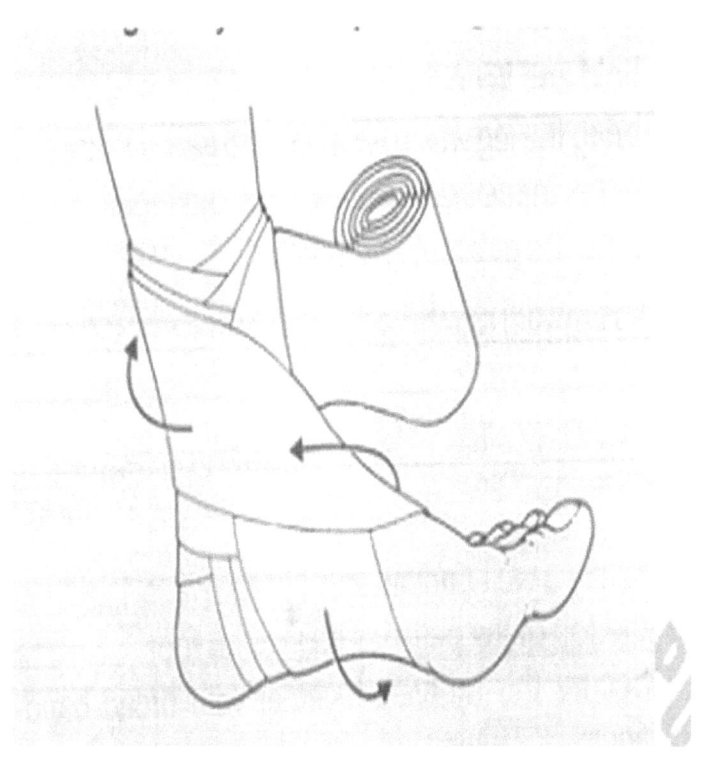

Fig. 20 Bandaging of sprain ankle

SECTION SIX

Burns

Burns are injuries to skin and other tissues caused by fire, thermal, radiation, chemical, or electric contact.Fire accident can cause great damage to life and properties. Children are the most vulnerable group to burn. Burns that occur around the mouth and nose or on the face are more dangerous and can cause death.Burns injuries cause about 3000 death per year in the US alone.

Causes of burns:

1.   Thermal burns from source like Fire, boiled water, steam, boiled oil and milk etc;

2.   Radiation burns like Sunburn and Ultraviolet radiation

3.   Electric generation heat and thunder accidents

4.   Different chemicals burns like strong acid and alkalis

Effect of the burn accident:

Immediate effects

1.   Burns and wounds of the body;

2.   Severe pain

3.   Hypovolemia due to reduction of body fluid from the wound

4. Difficulty in breathing due to suffocation from smoke, severe burns around the throat and face.

5.   Shock and unconsciousness.

Delayed effects/hazards:

1.   Infections of the wound, septicemia, and high fever

2.   Disability

3.   Scar formation

4.   Contracture

5.   Tetanus infection

Classification of burns:

Burns are classified into three levels based on the depth or degree of skin damage. These are:-

1.   First-degree burn

2.   Second-degree burn

3.   Third-degree burn

Characteristics of the first-degree burn:

1. Redness or discoloration.

2. Swelling and pain.

3. Healing is rapidly

Characteristics of Second-degree burn:

1. Greater in-depth than first degree burns

2. Redness and mottled appearance

3. Present of blisters

4. Severe pain

5. Swelling

6. The potential for infection.

Characteristic of third-degree burn:

1. Deep tissue distraction

2. White appearance

3. No pain and blisters

4. Complete loss of all layers of skin.

This type of burn results in severe disability and death.

First aid measures for burn injury

If the victim has burned with fire apply cold applications, immerse the burned area in cold water or role the burned person on the ground.

1. Cover with a water soaked thick cloth or blanket and put out the fire.

2. If the accident is from the electric source, quickly disconnect the electric meter or checkpoint, or use rope wooden stick, dried cloth, to disconnect it.

3. Move the victim away from the accident place to avoid further injury.

4. Loosen and remove burned dresses and lay down the victim on his back and let him breathe fresh air.

5.   Ensure that no foreign objects have entered and blocked the passage of the respiratory system

6.   If the victim is not breathing adequately, initiate mouth to mouth artificial respiration

7.   Check the wound to determine the size and the degree of burn

Measures for 1st-degree burn:

1.   Apply cold-water application or submerge the burned area in cold water

2.   If the wound is small, clean daily the area with boiled cold water cover it with the clean cloth to prevent contact with flies.

3.   If the wound located is in a joint, immobilize the joint area until the wound is cured

4.   If the wound is from boiled water, chemical (acid) take out his/her dress and cover it with the clean cloth.

First aid of 2nd and 3rd-degree burn:-

1.   Cover the wound with clean cloth

2. If the victim is conscious, his respiratory parts such as mouth, nose, and throat are free from the burn injury and gives him frequently plenty copies of liquid such as ORS or similar solution.

3.   Prepare the solution from eight teaspoons of sugar, one spoon salt in one liter of boiled cold water.

4.   If the victim is a child below two years give it one spoon every two minutes and if the child

144

is over two years give it with a cup or glass in the small amount every two minutes. The victim or his family should get tetanus toxoid vaccine

5.   Refer the victim to the nearest hospital.

6.   Take the victims immediately to a nearby health facility present with the following signs:

(a). First degree burn with sizeable area;

(b). 2nd and 3rd-degree burns;

(c).If the victim is drowsy, restless and has breathing problem;

(d) If the victim has burns on his face, eye, extremities,

(e) Joints and around genital organs;

If the source of the burn is electrical, chemical or thunder

145

(f)If the patient has chronic disease such as epilepsy, diabetes etc.; and

(g) If the burn accident is on elderly persons or children,

Education on preventive measures:

1.   Educating on the consequence of severe burns and training on fire fighting techniques.

2. Education to prevent using harmful foreign substances on the burned area.

3. Less frequent touching of the wound, or moving joints

4.   Identify the causes of the burn accident and have the appropriate

knowledge to the family and the community.

Measure to prevent burns

1. Keep all outreach of items such as matches, burning lamp, and candles

2. Prepare and place stoves and other cooking installations in a safe way that the children cannot reach.

3. Keep away from fire inflammable materials and don't' come with materials such as nylon close to a fireplace.

4. Smokers should not smoke inside a house and if they must smoke, give them strict advice to put off the burning leftover cigarette.

Poison

Accidental poisoning result in many emergencies visit and a few deaths. Any substance that, is dose-related which may result from exposure to an excess amount of normally not- toxic substances.if taken into the body in sufficient quantity, can cause temporary or permanent damage.Quickly, take the poisoned to the hospital or health center immediately.

General principle of poisoning first aid

Any contact with a substance that may result from tin toxicity, the symptom may differ, but the common syndrome may indicate classes of the poison. Most treatments are supportive with the specific antidote.

Assess the extent of danger depends upon

1. The quantity and type of poison
2. The age of the victim
3. Whether the victim vomits
4. Where the accident takes place and time

There are different causes of poisoning

1. Acids
2. Insecticides
3. Alkalis
4. Drugs are given for allergy (antihistamines)
5. Aspirin overdose in children
6. Sedatives
7. Iron

8. Mercury and lead

9. Paraffin, and petrol (Gasoline)

General signs and symptoms

1. Nausea

2. Vomiting

3. Severe abdominal pain

4. Change in consciousness

5. Change in vital signs

6. Change in pupils color

Poisons can enter into the body either accidentally or intentionally through

1. Ingestion by mouth

2. Inhalation by breathing

3. Absorption through the skin or through contact with poisonous by sprays, pesticide, and insecticides

4. Injection into the skin as the result of bites from animal, insects, poisonous fish or by syringe.

Steps to treatment of poison

1.   Remove the poison from the body
2.   Identify the particular poison antidote
3.   Treat symptoms
4.   Provide comfort and confidence

How to remove poison from the body

1.   induce victim to vomit it
2.   Give plenty of tap water.
3.   If it is a child give them syrup or water.
4.   Repeat the procedure
5.   Refer the victim if it is not improving

Do not induce vomiting if the poison e.g. paraffin or kerosene.

Do not make the victim vomit if unconscious.For poisoning by acid, give alkali, anti-acids. Poisoning can prevent by labeling drug container clearly and keeping them out the reach of children.

SECTION SEVEN

Bites and stings

Bites and stings cause the more than 100 death per year in the US alone. Bites are common and occasionally cause the significant morbidity and disability, human and mammal's bites are common. In addition to tissue trauma, infection from biting organism's oral floras while human bite can transmit viral hepatitis and HIV.

A. *Snake Bite*

There about 3000 differences species of snakes in the world, but Rattlesnake account for the majority of almost all related death. Snake venoms are the minor polypeptide that acts enzymes with lethal properties on various body organs.

Signs and symptoms

1.   Disturbed vision due neurotoxin
2.   Nausea or vomiting

3.   Two puncture wounds with sharp pain and local swelling

4.   Symptoms and sign of shock

5.   Sweating and salivation in advanced stages of venom reaction

First aid management snake bites

1.   Lay the victim down and advise not to move

2.   Avoid exertion and reassures the victim

3.   Immobilized the affected part and keep it below the level of the heart

4.   Constrictive clothing should be removed

5.   Wipe the wound of venom

6.   Apply firm tourniquet just above the bite

7.   This tourniquet must remove in 15 minutes if you are sure that anti-venom has been injected and you cannot get the victim to a hospital in time.

If there is no anti-venom do the following:

1.   Tie a cord tightly around the limb just above the bite.Using a razor blade or a clean knife make a cut 1 cm deep

2.   Use your mouth to Suck the liquid which is coming out of the wound

3.   Continue to suck and dispose of for 5-10 minutes

4.   Loosen the cord around the patient's limb

5.   Disinfect the wound

6.   Refer to the hospital for anti- venom

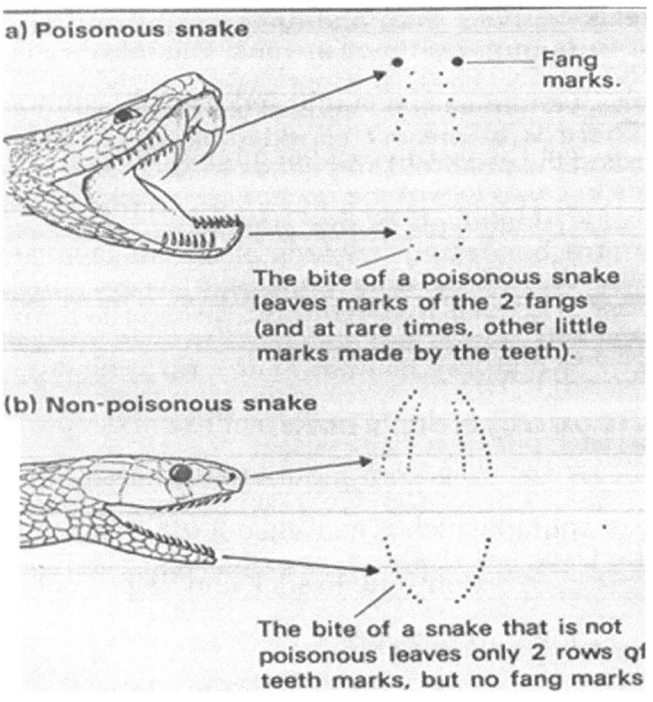

a) Poisonous snake

Fang marks.

The bite of a poisonous snake leaves marks of the 2 fangs (and at rare times, other little marks made by the teeth).

(b) Non-poisonous snake

The bite of a snake that is not poisonous leaves only 2 rows of teeth marks, but no fang marks

Fig .11. Snake bite

bite

injection.

B. Dog bite

Rabies is a sickness due to an infection from mammalian usually a rabies dog, cat, fox, wolf, and bats.The organism grows in the animal's nerves, may develop the disease, if the saliva enters a wound or scratch on a human being.

Characteristics of a rabid dog.

1. Difficulty in swallowing food
2. Rarely bite
3. Is lethargic and lazy
4. Hides itself
5. Does not want food, but swallows, pieces of wood stone slowly
6. Barks in an unusual way and never stop barking when it start
7. Saliva runs out from its mouth

First aid management of dog bites

1.   Immediately clean the wound with soap and water

2.   Cover the wound with dressing ointment/powders

3.   Find out if anyone knows the dog that bit the patient

4.   If the dog was known, ask its owner to watch the dog carefully for lodges and to let you know it shows any of the above characteristics in that time

5.   Observe, during that time, it begins to show any of the above characteristics.

6.   If above characteristics is confirmed, then get the dog killed

7. Send the victim to hospital or Health Center immediately for anti-rabies vaccination

Convulsion (fit)

When somebody has a sudden jerking movement and which cannot be controlled it is called fit or convulsion.It usually occurs due to the nervous excitation by toxins.

Signs and symptoms

1. uncontrolled jerking movements
2. Unconsciousness, not oriented to the environment place and time

Management of convulsion

1. Keep the airway clear and lie the victim on one side
2. Remove any clothes which are too tight around the neck

3.   Protect the victim from biting his tongue by putting tongue depressor in the mouth

4.   Record vital signs and time of fit

5.   Prevent victim from injury and fractures

6.   Educate the victim and the family to go to health center or a hospital for further investigation and management

SECTION EIGHT

Eye, Ear and Nose Injury

Injury to the eye

The eyes are delicate, they can be affected easily, therefore; immediate help should is required.

Signs and symptoms

1. Pain inside the eye

2. Cut around the eyeball

3. Different between left and right vision

4. Sight   decreases on acuity

5. Inflammation and infection

161

Management of the eye injury

1.   A very light covering dressing applied to an injured eyes

2.   Do not apply too much pressure

3.   Reassure the patient

4.   If no improvement in few days, Refer the victim to the nearest hospital

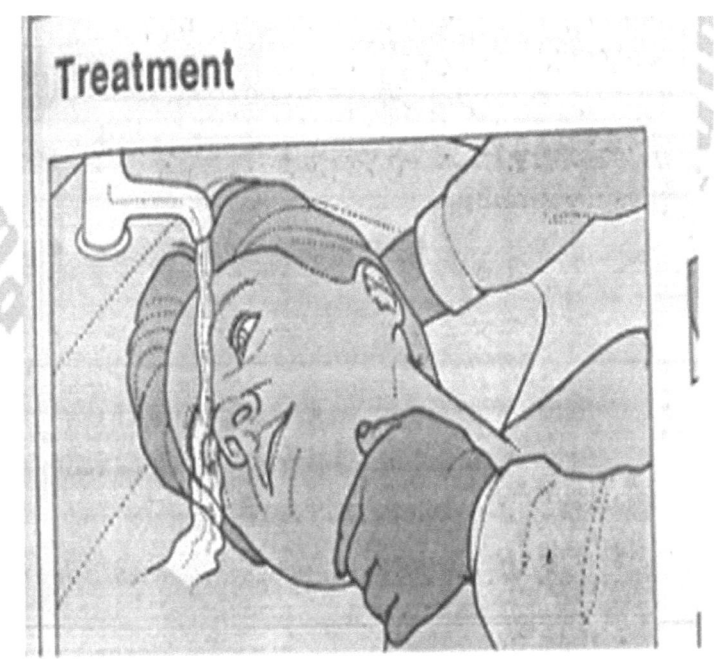

Hold the affected side of the eye

Fig. 21 removing foreign body in the
eye

Foreign bodies in the eyes

A foreign body can be dust, ash, particles of sands, or small fly.Often you can remove foreign from the eyes by flooding it with taped warm water.

If it does not work:

Instruct the victim not to rub his eyes, while the victim is looking up; gently draw the lower lid down and out.If the foreign body is seen on the lower lid remove it with moistened cotton wool or the corner of a clean handkerchief,

If it does not:

1.   Stand at front of the patient

2.   Carefully place a smooth match stick at the base lid and pull and turn it inside out over the match stick

3.   Remove the foreign body with wisp of Cottonwood

4.   you should not try to remove a foreign body from the eyeball with fingers

5.   If an acid or alkali gets into the eye, this can be very dangerous hence, flood the eye with running water for several minutes.Hold the affected side of the eye

Ear problems

Bleeding from the ear

Bleeding from the ear may be due to fractured skull

1.   Cover the ear with a clean material (sterile if available) dressing.

2.   Do not plug the ear with cotton wool

3.   Do not put in any drops

4. Refer the victim to the nearest health heath

Foreign body in the ear

1. Turn the patient's head to the affected part of the ear so that the foreign body may drop out due to gravity.

2. If it is an insect enters inside the ear, direct torch- light to the ear- the insect may follow the light and come out of the ear.

If this does not succeed

3. Pour in taped warm water, the insect may float out

4. If neither this treatment is successful, refer the client to the next health facility.

Bleeding from the Nose

1.   Instruct the patient to pinch the lower part of his nose firmly for 10 minutes, while breathing through his mouth

2.   Loosen tight clothing around victim's neck

3.   Tell the victim not to blow his nose for several hours

4.   If bleeding persists, refer the patient to the next health facility.

Foreign body in the nose

In an adult, the foreign body may enter the nose by accident, but most

167

common in children who insert a pea or a bean into their noses.

Do not attempt to remove it, refer to the next health facility.

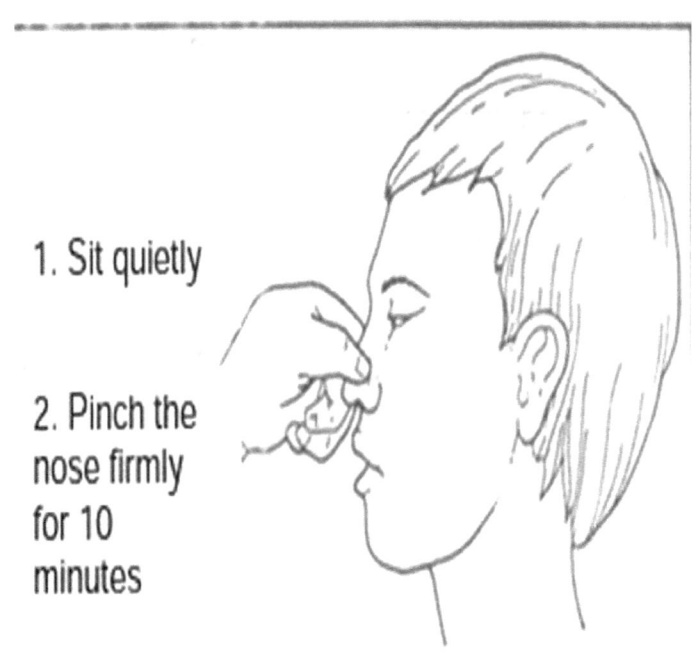

1. Sit quietly

2. Pinch the nose firmly for 10 minutes

Fig 22 How to stop a nosebleeding

1.   If the foreign body is either beans, peas, avoid putting water or any fluid

2.   Sit quietly

3.   Pinch the nose firmly for 10 minutes

Diarrhea

If a patient has over three frequent/subsequent loose stool in a day, it is called diarrhea.When an individual loses much fluid from the body due to diarrhea and vomiting, it is likely that he becomes unconscious and or dies.

Causes of diarrhea and vomiting:

1.   Food poisoning

2.   Intestinal parasites

Emerging adverse consequences:

1.   Depletion of body fluids

2. Unconsciousness

3. Kidneys failure

4. Malnourishment and dehydration

5. Death may occur, if untreated in time.

Signs of dehydration

1. Excessive loss of body fluids

2. Body debilitation and loss of weight

3. Dryness of the mouth or tongue, sunken eyeballs, eye drops, and sunken fontanel, in children

4. Dry and wrinkled skin, and when the skin on the stomach is stretched up with fingers and let down, it remains as wrinkled

5. Reduced amount of urine are observed

171

6. Shock and unconsciousness.

First aid measures diarrhea and vomiting

1. Ensure that there are no adverse signs that are usually precipitated by diarrhea and vomiting such as:

2. Sunken eyeballs, wrinkled skin, restlessness; and unconsciousness; and in children, continuous vomiting after taking fluids, shivering etc.

3. Prepare ORS in one liter of boiled and cold water.If ORS is not available to prepare homemade solution as follows.

4. Mix eight spoon of sugar, with half a spoon salt in one liter (three normal beer bottles) of boiled cold water.If available, add half a glass of orange or banana juice into the solution

5.   The ORS or home-made solution is prepared for an adult.Therefore, he must take the fluid in the small amount every five minutes. If the one-liter solution is not finished in 24 hours, prepare and give a new/fresh solution in the following day.In addition frequently provide the victim soup, rice-water, gruel/oatmeal (an adult can take daily up to three liters of fluid)

6.   For children give ORS or a solution mix of eight spoons of sugar and half spoon of salt in one liter of boiled cold water or the mix of 2 times rice flour or corn or wheat or smashed potato in one liter of water and boiled for 5-7 minutes.Feed children after it is properly cooled in the following manner.

7.   Children 2 months to 2 years old must get 50-100 milliliters (1 or 2 cups),

a maximum of 500 milliliters in one day (one spoon every 2 minutes)

8.   Children 2-10 years old must get 100-200 milliliters or 2-4 cups of ORS or home-made solution after every diarrhea episode the child can take up to one liter of the solution

9.   If the victim is over 10 years old, give the fluid until satisfied.

10.   If the victim vomits the fluid, wait for about 10 minutes, and give one spoon of the solution every three minutes;

11.   If it the child, frequently breastfeed the victim and add in the small amount other supplementary foods such as gruel/oatmeals every 10 minutes.

12.   Continue the supplementary feeding for about two weeks after diarrhea ceased.

The Rationale of the referral

1.   Persistent vomiting after taking fluids

2.   If the diarrhea is stained with blood and the victim has high fever

3.   If the vomiting is accompanied by sign such as tenderness and severe cramp of the stomach

4.   If diarrhea continues for 3 consecutive days, in children and 4 days in adults without improvement.

Measures were taken after first-aid assistance

1.   Explain the causes of diarrhea and vomiting'

2.   Observe in the presence of precipitating factors in the household, such as the maintenance of house cleanliness and personal hygiene

3.   water source usage, the handling of food and feeding practices.Based on the findings educate the household or the community with demonstrations.

Preventive Measures

1.   Demonstrate to the household on the importance of washing hands with soap and water, or with sand and water etc.before eating

2.   Feed children supplementary food and milk with cup and spoon or breastfeed instead of bottle feeding

3.   Keep children in clean areas and keep them always away from dirty area

176

4.   Don't feed on unclean and unprotected food stuff

5.   Use always latrines and toilets

6.   Maintain good personal hygiene and clean environment.

Diseases Characterized By Fever

When body's temperature is too hot than normal range (above 37.5 oc) he has a fever.However, fever itself is not an illness, but a sign of many different illnesses.

Common diseases that manifested with fever

1.   Yellow fever

2.   Typhus, Relapsing fever etc

3.   Typhoid

4.   Meningitis'

5.   Influenza

6.   Malaria

Adverse consequences of febrile illness

1.   Mental confusion, unconsciousness

2.   Reduction of body fluid

3.   Convulsion(fit)

4.   High fever may result in brain damage, paralysis, hypotension, dysfunction of kidneys, inability to hear, speak, and liver damage.

First-aid Measures for febrile condition

1.   Cover with or put a light dress on the victim.If the victim is a child, cover it with light cloth and carry it in your arms

2.   Replace fluids lost by profuse sweating give frequently the victim,

soup, gruel oatmeal, if the victim is a child, give frequently breast-milk

3. Put cloth soaked in lukewarm water on the chest, face, and abdomen to bring down the fever

4. Ensure perhaps the presence of convulsion, chillness, vomiting, diarrhea, meningitis etc

5. If the area is in the tropic malaria region and the fever has lasted for at least two days, give the victim malaria treatment according to the guidelines on malaria.

6. If the victim has not improved three days after he got the malaria treatment and if he has signs and symptoms such as vomiting, diarrhea, meningitis, jaundiced eyes, convulsion, inability to breathe, rapid and intermittent breathing, dyspnea, no

179

urination after drinks, mental confusion, unconscious etc.

7. if the locality is not malaria and the cause of the fever is unknown, bring the victim immediately to a nearby health facility for treatment.

8. If the victim is a child and has not improved with first-aid treatment, take him rapidly to the next health facility

9. Consult health facility to find out whether the cause of the fever is or not an infectious disease

10. Assess if a similar illness is observed in the same community, follow and register if the number of cases is rising.Then report and solicit support from the nearby health facility

11. Health education on the causes and preventive measures of the illness.

12.   When the cause is identified, treat accordingly or refer when necessary because meningitis and cerebral malaria are a serious condition to refer soon.

Preventive measures

1.   Clear all mosquito breeding places such as water collections, ditches etc

2.   Undertake insecticide residual house spraying

3.   Advise households to use insecticide-treated nets

4.   Avoid overcrowding

5.   Maintain hygiene personal and environmental hygiene

6.   Houses must have windows and the windows must be kept open

181

7. Allow cross ventilation of air through windows and doors in prisons, schools and in public meeting places

8. If there is any disease exists in the community report to the nearby health facility and in the meantime undertake a survey or assessment of the situation

9. If the number of cases increases, advise the community to stop gathering and in the meantime solicit and organize for vaccination programmed.

Signs and symptoms

1. Unconsciousness and delirium

2. Convulsion

3. Foaming saliva at the mouth

4. The white part of the eyeball becomes visible

5. When the convulsion subsides, the victim gradually becomes

conscious,but the victim is weak and dizzy.

Adverse consequences fever

1.   Depletion of oxygen in brain, dysfunction, and retardation of the brain

2.   The victim may suffer head damage, wound, body burns etc.during the attack; and Perhaps death.

First aid measures for febrile convulsion

1.   Remove the victim from potentially dangerous site to prevent him from further accident or injury while in convulsion

2.   Remove nearby dangerous objects to avoid the further accident, Loosen tight dress, necktie, belt etc.

3.   Lie the victim on his side to prevent the biting of his/her tongue, insert splint of wood wrapped by stripes of cloth in between his/her teeth

4.   Clean the foaming fluid coming out through the victim' mouth

5.   Keep him laid down on his side until jerking is over. When the jerking is over, bring him immediately to a nearby hospital

6.   Understand the cause of the sudden illness, and if the victim was already on drugs, advise and educate him to take medicine regularly.

7.   Also, keep record of the victim and follow him and advise him not to come near fire, or to stay always where there are people

8.   The victim should refrain from crossing deep rivers or climb high trees.

184

AUTHOBIOGRAPHY

Philip Kabcy was born in Oxford, Mississippi, to Dr. Billy Collin, a Professor of molecular physiology and biophysics the University of Southern Mississippi. He graduated from a college of health science; the University of California in 1953.He became a consultant in accident and emergency medicine in 1966.

Philip has over 40 years experience in trauma, burn and plastic surgery.He is a recipient of the collegiate teaching award and is currently the course director for Center disaster control at

185

University.Philip received his Ph.D. in hazard prevention from the University of California at Berkeley.His research interest is focused on the molecular gene therapy.

Philip K. PhD

www.ingramcontent.com/pod-product-compliance
Lightning Source LLC
Chambersburg PA
CBHW030444290526
45786CB00001B/430